I0439283

Dash Diet For Beginners:

Healthy Dieting Tips

By

Debra Helton

ISBN-13: 978-1495921315

Table of Contents

Dash Diet For Beginners: Healthy Dieting Tips

By Debra Helton

Introduction

Dash diet refers to dietary approaches to stop hypertension. As its name implies, Dash diet is a diet that's aimed for the purpose of controlling hypertension and reducing its attack on people. Hypertension is a no-joke condition that attacks almost all people, even people as young as 30 years old. Hypertension can lead to stroke and death if ignored and not controlled, which is why this is considered a serious condition that requires your attention.

With the increasing number of hypertension victims nowadays, people need to watch what they are eating because usually, it is the food that people eat that is the main cause of hypertension. Most of the foods consumed by people nowadays are either fatty or salty and most of the time, people consume too much of these foods. So, for the purpose of controlling hypertension, reduce its threat and reduce the number of hypertension-related deaths, the Dash diet was created. In fact, the Dash diet is highly recommended for all hypertension victims and for those people who want to prevent hypertension from knocking into their lives.

But before you rush into Dash diet, it is a must to get to know what type of diet you are going into first. What are the things you should expect from Dash diet? What are the things you should not expect? What foods are you recommended to eat and what foods are you advised to avoid in this diet? Is this diet really what hypertension victims need? This book Dash Diet For Beginners: Healthy Dieting Tips discusses all about Dash diet and will try to answer all questions that most people ask about it.

Chapter 1. The Principles of Dash Diet

For beginners, it is a must to know the principles of Dash diet first before going into this type of diet. The principles of Dash diet will get you informed about what Dash diet is all about so you will know what to expect when you go Dash.

Dash diet is a diet of fruits and vegetables. This does not mean that Dash diet is a vegetarian diet though, but it only means that this diet is high in fruits and vegetables to get all the potassium, magnesium and fiber that your body needs. Fiber is a very good carrier of wastes, including fats, to be excreted out of the body.

Dash diet is a low-sodium diet. Sodium is one of the main culprits that trigger hypertension especially too much intake of it. In Dash diet, the consumption of low sodium foods is advised. This encourages people to reduce the use of salt on their food no matter what they are cooking as well as avoid salty foods.

Dash diet is a low-fat dairy diet but a high calcium diet. Hypertension victims can still consume dairy products because these are main sources of calcium and hypertension victims need to increase their calcium intake. But in Dash diet, low-fat dairy products are recommended. Fat is one main culprit that trigger hypertension as well and reducing the intake of fats by consuming low-fat dairy products can help reduce the risk of hypertension.

Dash diet is a diet of low-saturated fat consumption. Saturated fats are the main culprit that can raise cholesterol levels and trigger hypertension. These fats are fats that lurk inside the body especially in your blood. With this, Dash diet is a diet that encourages low consumption of these saturated fats or foods that are sources of saturated fats, in order to stop hypertension.

Chapter 2. Foods Recommended in Dash Diet

Like any other diet plans, there are also certain foods that Dash diet recommends. Knowing the foods that are recommended in Dash diet will help you gain awareness of the foods that are right for you especially if you have hypertension. This will give you awareness that not all foods out there are good for you. And abiding by the recommended foods in Dash diet will help you easily stop hypertension and control the condition instead of hypertension controlling you. Here are some of the foods in various categories recommended in a Dash diet:

Fruits and Vegetables: Not all fruits and vegetables are recommended in Dash diet. But these fruits and vegetables are: Apple, banana, berries, bell pepper, cabbage, broccoli, cauliflower, corn, carrots, grapes, lemon, mushroom, lettuce, onions, pear, pineapple, raisins, squash, potatoes and sprouts.

Meat and Seafood: Although meat, especially red meat and seafood are advised to be taken moderately, it does not mean that you cannot consume these foods in Dash diet. In the meat and seafood category, Dash diet recommends: Beef, Turkey, fish like salmon, chicken, as well as shrimp.

Bread and Grains: Not all types of grains are recommended in a Dash diet as well as not all breads are good for hypertension victims. When it comes to bread and grains, these are recommended in a Dash diet: brown rice, whole wheat bread, tortillas, pasta, and cereal, barley, oats, and wild rice.

Nuts and Seeds: Nuts and seeds are also recommended in a Dash diet but the most common foods under this category that are highly recommended are: pecans, almonds, peanuts, pumpkin seeds, cashews, and walnuts.

Dairy: Dairy products are excellent sources of calcium; however, in a Dash diet the consumption of dairy products should be limited to certain dairy products such as: reduced-fat cheese like cottage cheese, non-fat milk, sour cream, margarine and some yogurt.

All these foods contain all the nutrients you need and at the same time, helping you control hypertension.

Chapter 3. Foods Not Recommended in a Dash Diet

If there are foods recommended in a Dash diet, there are also foods that are either not recommended, highly discouraged in a Dash diet or foods that are advised to be taken in very small amounts if you are on a Dash diet. The importance of getting to know these foods is you will know what you're not supposed to eat while you are still trying to control your hypertensive condition. Avoiding these foods or avoiding the high consumption of these foods can help you successful control hypertension and be successful in your Dash diet goal.

Meat and Poultry: You are not altogether restricted to eat meat in Dash diet but you are advised not to consume meats that are canned such as: luncheon meat, smoked meat like barbecue, etc. There should also be a limit to consuming poultry products like egg, especially the egg yolk because of its high cholesterol levels.

Condiments: While condiments make your meals special and extra delicious, in Dash diet, you should avoid condiments such as: ketchup, soy sauce, salt and salted sauces. If you may need to use condiments for your meals, as long as you can guarantee they are low-fat and low-salt condiments, you can add them on your meals.

Packed and processed foods. In a Dash diet, there should be no room for packed and processed foods because they already contain preservatives and Trans fats that could increase your blood cholesterol levels, you should avoid: canned pickles and processed and preserved sausages, etc.

Cured foods: In a Dash diet you should also avoid cured foods such as: ham, buttered chicken, etc.

Sweets: In a dash diet, it is highly advised to avoid too much sweets or foods that contain too much sugar in them like: candy bars, ice cream, soft drinks, pies, etc.

Junk foods: In a dash diet, this is a no-no. Since dash diet is a low sodium diet, it is not only the salty condiments that you should avoid but also junk foods such as: salted popcorn, noodles, potato chips, etc. Junk foods are not only salty but they also contain a great deal of Trans fats that could be harmful for your hypertensive condition.

Chapter 4. Dash Diet Meal Plan

If you are on a Dash diet, it is a must to create and follow a Dash diet meal plan. A Dash diet meal plan will serve as your guide towards a successful Dash diet since you will have a reference as to what you should eat and how often certain foods should be consumed. A meal plan can help you avoid over eating the wrong foods and make sure that you are eating the right amount of good and highly recommended foods. Here is an example of a Dash diet meal plan in different food groups and information as to how often and how many servings are recommended in day.

Grains: Whether you consume grain foods for breakfast, lunch, snacks or dinner, grains should be eaten at least 6-8 servings a day. You can consume grains in different varieties such as whole wheat bread, cereals, and brown rice.

Vegetables: You should consume 4-5 servings of vegetables daily especially vegetables like broccoli, spinach, tomatoes, carrots, etc. Vegetables to consume should not be overcooked or if you can, eat them raw or in the form of juice.

Fruits: In a day, you should consume 4-5 servings of fruits. You can choose to consume it in the form of juice, eat it directly or whip up a salad of fruits like apples, pineapples, peaches, strawberries, and a lot more.

Dairy: You should only consume 2-3 servings of dairy products daily. It is either you drink milk for breakfast, snack and dinner or substitute milk with yogurt with cheese sandwich for snacks. Just make sure all the dairy products you consume in a day are fat-free.

Lean Meat: Meat should be taken in moderation especially if you are eating pork and chicken meat and make sure you only eat the lean part of the meat. 6 servings of lean meat in a day or less is enough to give you your daily dose of protein and magnesium.

Seeds and Nuts: You can incorporate nuts in your snack because they are rich sources of protein and magnesium too. 4-5 servings per week are enough especially if you are also eating lean meat daily. Make your nuts and seeds a mix of almonds, lentils, or even peanut butter.

Fats and oils: Fats and oils should only be consumed in moderation and depending on your food sources. 2-3 servings of fats and oils daily are enough and make sure they are friendly fat sources like margarine and vegetable oil.

Sweets: You can also treat yourself with sweets in dash diet but should be limited. At least 5 servings of sweets like candy and ice cream per week is enough if you cannot avoid it altogether.

Chapter 5. Dash Diet Meal Plan Examples

1. Breakfast

The body goes through a long fast when it sleeps through the night; you do not eat for more than 6 to 8 hours a day therefore your DASH breakfast should be heavy to nourish you after your fast and to keep you till your mid-morning snack all the while following a strict diet that will maintain your blood pressure and blood sugar levels.

Sample meal plan 1 – strawberry jam on a slice of whole wheat bread, oatmeal drizzled with apple sauce, a banana and fruit juice. The DASH diet recommends adding more fruits and whole grains in your diet for a hearty supply of fiber. Strawberry jam, apples sauce and bananas will keep you full longer plus whole wheat bread is a great source of fiber.

You may slightly toast your wheat bread while add more fruits to your oatmeal. You have a choice on what kind of fruit juice you want to drink.

Plan 2 – blueberry muffins with a light butter spread, skim milk and a slice of cantaloupe. Blueberries and cantaloupes are sweet and tasty plus contain vitamins and minerals to boost the immune system. Choose light butter spread but use only one pat. Skim milk contains calcium and minerals and is low in fat to keep you trim and fit.

Plan 3 - wheat cereal with skim milk, chunks of bananas and strawberries and a cup of fruity yoghurt. Wheat cereal is an excellent source of fiber along with fruits in this meal plan. Fruits like bananas and strawberries contain high amounts of potassium which is good for the heart.

Plan 4 – light tuna in oil over wheat bread, fruit medley and cream. About 3 ounces of tuna (a small can) contains amazing amounts of protein and omega 3s that contributes to a healthy heart. Place this over toasted wheat bread and drizzle with oil for a hearty and tasty breakfast treat. Choose fruits in season like apples, papayas, berries or pineapples and top your fruits with light cream.

Plan 5 – English muffins with light cream cheese, skim milk and frozen berries. Choose freshly made muffins but make sure you top it only a pat of light cream cheese. Frozen berries could be blueberries, blackberries or strawberries or a combination.

2. Lunch

Your body needs energy especially during mid-morning when you feel sleepier instead of being pumped up to perform at work or do activities at home. The DASH diet offers a wide variety of foods to eat even when you need to maintain your blood pressure and blood sugar levels. The DASH diet may also be used for weight loss so these sample meal plans are not just healthy but are also satisfying to help you feel fuller till dinner time and prevent snacking on high calorie foods in the afternoon.

Sample meal plan 1 – turkey breast and Swiss cheese on whole wheat bread, veggies strips, frozen berries and ice tea. Turkey breast is a rich source of protein at 11% per 33g and 99.96mg potassium. A slice of Swiss cheese contains 31mg of potassium which is also good for the heart.

Plan 2 – tuna on whole wheat pita bread, steamed vegetables, a slice of cantaloupe or pineapple. A can of tuna (165g) contains 42.1g or 84% of your daily protein needs. Whole wheat pita bread is a rich fiber source together with steamed veggies of your choice. Fruits like cantaloupes and pineapples are perfect sources of vitamin C and studies show that ample intake of vitamin C each day could lower a person's risk of suffering from coronary heart disease.

Plan 3 – fried chicken breast minus the skin, coleslaw, baby carrots and baby corn and sugar-free Jell-O. Remove the skin and marinate chicken in salt, pepper, minced garlic and soy sauce. Deep fry in palm oil. Veggies in coleslaw, baby carrots and corn are great sources of fiber, minerals and vitamins.

Plan 4 – chicken in light mayo salad, a small dinner roll, a banana and pineapple juice. Boil chicken breast and when it is done, prepare the salad by flaking chicken and adding light mayo dressing plus a little salt and pepper to taste.

Plan 5 – sardine in light oil over whole wheat bread, side vegetable salad and a slice of melon. Sardine is a great source of phosphorous and as a high level of good fat which is essential in making the heart healthy. Choose crisp veggies like romaine lettuce, carrots, red peppers and tomatoes plus add hard-boiled egg slices and drizzle with light mayonnaise.

3. Dinner

Dinner is best enjoyed with family but this does not mean you have to skip following the DASH diet plan. Foods served should help maintain blood pressure and ideal blood sugar levels and follow the DASH guidelines on serving more fruits, vegetables, low fat and nonfat foods, whole grains, lean meats, poultry, fish and food sources that are rich in heart-healthy fats.

Sample meal plan 1 – tilapia seared with light butter, baby carrots and corn, strawberry flavored gelatin. Tilapia is a meaty fish with a sweet and tender flesh perfect for grilling, frying and searing. Tilapia has high protein content and minerals that are needed for a healthy heart. The trick to searing tender fish is to heat the pan or grille to maximum while the fish is at room temperature. Season the fish with a bit of salt and pepper and then apply butter on each side. When the grille is hot enough, place the tilapia and then wait for about 5 minutes to turn.

Plan 2 – whole wheat spaghetti with tomatoes, mushrooms and light Swiss cheese, fruit salad with fruits in season and ice tea. Whole wheat noodles are perfect source of carbohydrates and fiber perfect for a healthy heart. Eating more fiber-rich foods will reduce your risk of suffering from conditions of the cardiovascular system.

Plan 3 – Crunchy vegetables dipped in homemade guacamole dip, grilled chicken, romaine lettuce salad with Italian dressing, sugar-free Jell-O. Guacamole is made of avocadoes which are considered one of the healthiest foods that is also heart friendly. Make your own guacamole dip by blending avocado slices, tomatoes, chives, cilantro and onions in a food processor. Prepare crunchy veggies slices like carrots, red bell peppers, cucumbers, etc.

Plan 4 – roasted turkey breast, side salad with Italian dressing drizzle, an apple and fruit juice. Turkey breast contains amazing amounts of protein and minerals while apples also contain vitamins and minerals for a healthy and fit body and heart.

Plan 5 – grilled salmon, baked potato, several strips of steamed asparagus and frozen yoghurt. Salmon is one of the healthiest foods; prepare your salmon with a little bit of salt, pepper and freshly squeezed lemon.

4. Snacks

The DASH diet suggests eating more fruits for snacks. Fruits in season can be made into a wide variety of snack foods like smoothies, fruit preserves, fruit candies, dried fruits and fruit ice cream. There are more ways to prepare fruits for snacks and you will never run out of ways to serve fruits as a morning or afternoon snack.

The best fruits that you should always have at home are berries (strawberries, blueberries and blackberries), apples, papayas, melons, kiwis, nectarines and grapes. Keep small cups of berries in the freezer so you can eat them for snacks or as dessert. Other fruits may be tossed in a salad or drizzled with light cream just before serving.

Cheese is not just a breakfast food but small bits of cheese (cheddar, Swiss, etc.) may be placed in toasted wheat bread or low salt crackers for snacks. Pick light cheeses to reduce your sodium intake.

Nuts like Brazil nuts, peanuts, pecans, almonds, pistachios, cashews and so many more will make great snack foods but choose light nuts and unsalted ones. Nuts also make you feel fuller longer and have low calorie content. Place a handful of almonds nearby as you study or work. You may also place a handful in a resealable bag so you can take it as you commute.

Vegetables are perfect for snacks and the crispier the better. Choose veggies wisely and inspect the skin before slicing or dicing them. Dip them in light mayonnaise, salad dressing or light cheese.

Jell-O is light, delicious and filling. This may be a great snack that has very little calories. You can eat Jell-O as much as you want and as often as you like without having to worry about your weight. There are so many Jell-O flavors to choose from: lemon, lime, orange, strawberry, grape and plain. You may also eat Jell-O as dessert food for lunch, dinner and for breakfast.

Yoghurt is another snack that you can eat before lunch and before dinner. it is primarily a dairy product but has amazing amounts of vitamins and minerals plus live microorganisms that will help restore gastrointestinal health. Yoghurt is also available in different flavors plus are easy to use and take along anywhere.

Chapter 5. Advantages of Dash Diet

Once you have start trying out Dash diet, you will realize that it is indeed advantageous because of the many benefits it can give you and your hypertension such as:

Lower blood pressure or controlled hypertension. Since you will be eating only the recommended foods in a Dash diet, you can control your hypertension already. You can prevent the increase of your blood pressure by lowering it to normal all the time.

Lower LDL cholesterol levels.LDL cholesterol or bad cholesterol levels are dangerous for the heart. It is not only a trigger point of hypertension but it can also lead to cardiovascular diseases. By eating only the right foods in a dash diet as well as eating with the right amount, you can greatly decrease bad cholesterol levels and save your heart.

Reduce the risk of stroke. Since you are lowering blood cholesterol levels through Dash diet, you also reduce your risk of stroke.

Reduce the risk of diabetes. In Dash diet, the consumption of sweets is advised to be avoided altogether or to limit your consumption of too much sweet. This then could help you reduce your risk of diabetes aside from controlling hypertension.

Reduce the risk of kidney diseases. High sodium diet is not only a trigger point of hypertension but it is also a great way to acquire kidney diseases like kidney stones. Through Dash diet, you can also save your kidney from diseases since it is a low-sodium diet.

Aids in weight loss. Dash diet may not be a sole contributor to weight loss. It cannot be considered as the ultimate weight loss solution as it is not created for weight loss. However, it can aid in weight loss too since some of the foods that contribute to weight gain are also limited or avoided in this diet.

Chapter 6. Possible Side Effects of Dash Diet

Another common question asked about Dash diet is whether it is safe and free from side effects or not. Normally, Dash diet is a really safe diet and is free from negative side effects. However, there are circumstances that may trigger the presence of side effects when you are on a Dash diet. It is important to be aware of these circumstances and side effects so that you can ensure you are safe before you start going Dash.

First, according to the principles of Dash diet, this is a high fiber diet. While this is a good thing as fiber has so many benefits for the body especially in excreting out unwanted fats and wastes, the intake of too much fiber can cause side effects such as diarrhea, bloating and gas. If fiber is also consumed without the aid of water, side effects such as constipation may be experienced. This is why it is a must to follow the recommended meal plan servings of fiber daily to reduce these side effects.

Another possible side effect of Dash diet is usually experienced by those who have abnormal kidney function.

If you have a healthy kidney function, you are exempted from this side effect but if you have impaired kidney function, hyperkalemia or the condition wherein there is high level of potassium in the blood may be experienced. Hyperkalemia is a serious condition because it can cause irregular heart beat so instead of being safe from cardiovascular disease because of Dash, the diet may prove to be a danger for you instead.

Conclusion

To sum up, hypertension is becoming one of the leading concerns of most people nowadays. A lot of people are already experiencing stroke and cardiovascular problems because of this. This is why, among the many types of diet plans being introduced nowadays, the DASH diet is made exclusively for hypertension control. Just like other diet plans out there, Dash diet may not be easy especially for beginners. It may not be easy to start and maintain especially if you are used to eating all the foods that you are required to let go once you are on a Dash diet. But once you realize just how serious hypertension is and how important it is to stop it through proper diet, Dash diet will just be a normal routine for you. You can even create your own Dash diet plan based on the foods you can eat.

However, because of some circumstances that could trigger the possible side effects of Dash diet, it is important to consult your doctor first before starting this diet.

Thank You Page

I want to personally thank you for reading my book. I hope you found information in this book useful and I would be very grateful if you could leave your honest review about this book. I certainly want to thank you in advance for doing this.